The Medical Health Checklist8

Copyright: Published in the United States by Rita L. Spears
Published March 2017

All rights reserved. No part of this publication may be reproduced, stored in retrieval system, copied in any form or by any means, electronic, mechanical, photocopying, recording or otherwise transmitted without written permission from the publisher. Please do not participate in or encourage piracy of this material in any way. You must not circulate this book in any format. Rita L. Spears *does not control or direct users' actions and is not responsible for the information or content shared, harm and/or actions of the book readers.*

ISBN-13: 978-1544794884

ISBN-10: 1544794886

Medical Release	
Patient's name	Date of Birth
Previous name	Social Security number

I request and authorize _____ to release healthcare information of The above named patient.		
Name		Address
City	State	Zip code
This request and authorization applies to _____		
Healthcare information relating to the following condition, treatment and dates: All healthcare information: Other: Yes: _____ No: _____		
I authorize the release of my STD/HIV/AIDS results whether negative or positive to the Above named person. Yes: _____ No: _____		
I authorize the release of any record regarding drug, alcohol or mental treatment to the Above named person.		
Patient Signature		Date Signed	
This authorization expires ninety days after it is issued.			

Medical Release

Patient's name	Date of Birth

Previous name	Social Security number

I request and authorize _____ to release healthcare information of
The above named patient.

Name	Address

City	State	Zip code

This request and authorization applies to _____

Healthcare information relating to the following condition, treatment and dates:
All healthcare information:
Other:
Yes: _____ No: _____

I authorize the release of my STD/HIV/AIDS results whether negative or positive to the
Above named person. Yes: _____ No: _____

I authorize the release of any record regarding drug, alcohol or mental treatment to the
Above named person.

Patient Signature		Date Signed	

This authorization expires ninety days after it is issued.

Medical Release

Patient's name	Date of Birth

Previous name	Social Security number

I request and authorize _____ to release healthcare information of
The above named patient.

Name	Address

City	State	Zip code

This request and authorization applies to _____

Healthcare information relating to the following condition, treatment and dates:
All healthcare information:
Other:
Yes: _____ No: _____

I authorize the release of my STD/HIV/AIDS results whether negative or positive to the
Above named person. Yes: _____ No: _____

I authorize the release of any record regarding drug, alcohol or mental treatment to the
Above named person.

Patient Signature		Date Signed	

This authorization expires ninety days after it is issued.

Medical Release	
Patient's name	Date of Birth
Previous name	Social Security number

I request and authorize _____ to release healthcare information of
The above named patient.

Name	Address

City	State	Zip code

This request and authorization applies to _____

Healthcare information relating to the following condition, treatment and dates:
All healthcare information:
Other:
Yes: _____ No: _____

I authorize the release of my STD/HIV/AIDS results whether negative or positive to the
Above named person. Yes: _____ No: _____

I authorize the release of any record regarding drug, alcohol or mental treatment to the
Above named person.

Patient Signature		Date Signed	

This authorization expires ninety days after it is issued.

Medical Release	
Patient's name	Date of Birth
Previous name	Social Security number

I request and authorize _____ to release healthcare information of The above named patient.		
Name		Address
City	State	Zip code
This request and authorization applies to _____		
Healthcare information relating to the following condition, treatment and dates: All healthcare information: Other: Yes: _____ No: _____		
I authorize the release of my STD/HIV/AIDS results whether negative or positive to the Above named person. Yes: _____ No: _____		
I authorize the release of any record regarding drug, alcohol or mental treatment to the Above named person.		
Patient Signature		Date Signed
This authorization expires ninety days after it is issued.		

Medical Release

Patient's name	Date of Birth

Previous name	Social Security number

I request and authorize _____ to release healthcare information of
The above named patient.

Name	Address

City	State	Zip code

This request and authorization applies to _____

Healthcare information relating to the following condition, treatment and dates:
All healthcare information:
Other:
Yes: _____ No: _____

I authorize the release of my STD/HIV/AIDS results whether negative or positive to the
Above named person. Yes: _____ No: _____

I authorize the release of any record regarding drug, alcohol or mental treatment to the
Above named person.

Patient Signature		Date Signed	

This authorization expires ninety days after it is issued.

Medical Release

Patient's name	Date of Birth

Previous name	Social Security number

I request and authorize _____ to release healthcare information of
The above named patient.

Name	Address

City	State	Zip code

This request and authorization applies to _____

Healthcare information relating to the following condition, treatment and dates:
All healthcare information:
Other:
Yes: _____ No: _____

I authorize the release of my STD/HIV/AIDS results whether negative or positive to the
Above named person. Yes: _____ No: _____

I authorize the release of any record regarding drug, alcohol or mental treatment to the
Above named person.

Patient Signature		Date Signed	

This authorization expires ninety days after it is issued.

Medical Release	
Patient's name	Date of Birth
Previous name	Social Security number
I request and authorize _____ to release healthcare information of The above named patient.	
Name	Address
City	State	Zip code
This request and authorization applies to _____	
Healthcare information relating to the following condition, treatment and dates: All healthcare information: Other: Yes: _____ No: _____	
I authorize the release of my STD/HIV/AIDS results whether negative or positive to the Above named person. Yes: _____ No: _____	
I authorize the release of any record regarding drug, alcohol or mental treatment to the Above named person.	
Patient Signature		Date Signed	
This authorization expires ninety days after it is issued.	

Medical Release	
Patient's name	Date of Birth
Previous name	Social Security number

I request and authorize _____ to release healthcare information of The above named patient.		
Name		Address
City	State	Zip code
This request and authorization applies to _____		
Healthcare information relating to the following condition, treatment and dates: All healthcare information: Other: Yes: _____ No: _____		
I authorize the release of my STD/HIV/AIDS results whether negative or positive to the Above named person. Yes: _____ No: _____		
I authorize the release of any record regarding drug, alcohol or mental treatment to the Above named person.		
Patient Signature		Date Signed	
This authorization expires ninety days after it is issued.		

Medical Release

Patient's name	Date of Birth

Previous name	Social Security number

I request and authorize _____ to release healthcare information of
The above named patient.

Name	Address

City	State	Zip code

This request and authorization applies to _____

Healthcare information relating to the following condition, treatment and dates:
All healthcare information:
Other:
Yes: _____ No: _____

I authorize the release of my STD/HIV/AIDS results whether negative or positive to the
Above named person. Yes: _____ No: _____

I authorize the release of any record regarding drug, alcohol or mental treatment to the
Above named person.

Patient Signature		Date Signed	

This authorization expires ninety days after it is issued.

Medical Release	
Patient's name	Date of Birth
Previous name	Social Security number

I request and authorize _____ to release healthcare information of
The above named patient.

Name	Address

City	State	Zip code

This request and authorization applies to _____

Healthcare information relating to the following condition, treatment and dates:
All healthcare information:
Other:
Yes: _____ No: _____

I authorize the release of my STD/HIV/AIDS results whether negative or positive to the
Above named person. Yes: _____ No: _____

I authorize the release of any record regarding drug, alcohol or mental treatment to the
Above named person.

Patient Signature		Date Signed	

This authorization expires ninety days after it is issued.

Medical Release

Patient's name	Date of Birth

Previous name	Social Security number

I request and authorize _____ to release healthcare information of
The above named patient.

Name	Address

City	State	Zip code

This request and authorization applies to _____

Healthcare information relating to the following condition, treatment and dates:
All healthcare information:
Other:
Yes: _____ No: _____

I authorize the release of my STD/HIV/AIDS results whether negative or positive to the
Above named person. Yes: _____ No: _____

I authorize the release of any record regarding drug, alcohol or mental treatment to the
Above named person.

Patient Signature		Date Signed	

This authorization expires ninety days after it is issued.

Medical Release	
Patient's name	Date of Birth
Previous name	Social Security number

I request and authorize _____ to release healthcare information of
The above named patient.

Name	Address

City	State	Zip code

This request and authorization applies to _____

Healthcare information relating to the following condition, treatment and dates:
All healthcare information:
Other:
Yes: _____   No: _____

I authorize the release of my STD/HIV/AIDS results whether negative or positive to the
Above named person. Yes: _____   No: _____

I authorize the release of any record regarding drug, alcohol or mental treatment to the
Above named person.

Patient Signature		Date Signed	

This authorization expires ninety days after it is issued.

Medical Release	
Patient's name	Date of Birth
Previous name	Social Security number
I request and authorize _____ to release healthcare information of The above named patient.	
Name	Address
City	State	Zip code

This request and authorization applies to _____
Healthcare information relating to the following condition, treatment and dates: All healthcare information: Other: Yes: _____ No: _____
I authorize the release of my STD/HIV/AIDS results whether negative or positive to the Above named person. Yes: _____ No: _____
I authorize the release of any record regarding drug, alcohol or mental treatment to the Above named person.

Patient Signature		Date Signed	
This authorization expires ninety days after it is issued.			

Medical Release

Patient's name	Date of Birth

Previous name	Social Security number

I request and authorize _____ to release healthcare information of
The above named patient.

Name	Address

City	State	Zip code

This request and authorization applies to _____

Healthcare information relating to the following condition, treatment and dates:
All healthcare information:
Other:
Yes: _____   No: _____

I authorize the release of my STD/HIV/AIDS results whether negative or positive to the
Above named person. Yes: _____   No: _____

I authorize the release of any record regarding drug, alcohol or mental treatment to the
Above named person.

Patient Signature		Date Signed	

This authorization expires ninety days after it is issued.

Medical Release	
Patient's name	Date of Birth
Previous name	Social Security number
I request and authorize _____ to release healthcare information of The above named patient.	
Name	Address
City	State	Zip code
This request and authorization applies to _____	
Healthcare information relating to the following condition, treatment and dates: All healthcare information: Other: Yes: _____ No: _____	
I authorize the release of my STD/HIV/AIDS results whether negative or positive to the Above named person. Yes: _____ No: _____	
I authorize the release of any record regarding drug, alcohol or mental treatment to the Above named person.	
Patient Signature		Date Signed	
This authorization expires ninety days after it is issued.	

Medical Release		
Patient's name		Date of Birth
Previous name		Social Security number
I request and authorize _____ to release healthcare information of The above named patient.		
Name		Address
City	State	Zip code
This request and authorization applies to _____		
Healthcare information relating to the following condition, treatment and dates: All healthcare information: Other: Yes: _____ No: _____		
I authorize the release of my STD/HIV/AIDS results whether negative or positive to the Above named person. Yes: _____ No: _____		
I authorize the release of any record regarding drug, alcohol or mental treatment to the Above named person.		
Patient Signature		Date Signed
This authorization expires ninety days after it is issued.		

Medical Release

Patient's name	Date of Birth

Previous name	Social Security number

I request and authorize _____ to release healthcare information of
The above named patient.

Name	Address

City	State	Zip code

This request and authorization applies to _____

Healthcare information relating to the following condition, treatment and dates:
All healthcare information:
Other:
Yes: _____   No: _____

I authorize the release of my STD/HIV/AIDS results whether negative or positive to the
Above named person. Yes: _____   No: _____

I authorize the release of any record regarding drug, alcohol or mental treatment to the
Above named person.

Patient Signature		Date Signed	

This authorization expires ninety days after it is issued.

Medical Release	
Patient's name	Date of Birth
Previous name	Social Security number

I request and authorize _____ to release healthcare information of
The above named patient.

Name	Address

City	State	Zip code

This request and authorization applies to _____

Healthcare information relating to the following condition, treatment and dates:
All healthcare information:
Other:
Yes: _____   No: _____

I authorize the release of my STD/HIV/AIDS results whether negative or positive to the
Above named person. Yes: _____   No: _____

I authorize the release of any record regarding drug, alcohol or mental treatment to the
Above named person.

Patient Signature		Date Signed	

This authorization expires ninety days after it is issued.

Medical Release	
Patient's name	Date of Birth
Previous name	Social Security number
I request and authorize _____ to release healthcare information of The above named patient.	
Name	Address
City	State	Zip code
This request and authorization applies to _____	
Healthcare information relating to the following condition, treatment and dates: All healthcare information: Other: Yes: _____ No: _____	
I authorize the release of my STD/HIV/AIDS results whether negative or positive to the Above named person. Yes: _____ No: _____	
I authorize the release of any record regarding drug, alcohol or mental treatment to the Above named person.	
Patient Signature		Date Signed	
This authorization expires ninety days after it is issued.	

Medical Release	
Patient's name	Date of Birth
Previous name	Social Security number

I request and authorize _____ to release healthcare information of The above named patient.

Name	Address

City	State	Zip code

This request and authorization applies to _____

Healthcare information relating to the following condition, treatment and dates:
All healthcare information:
Other:
Yes: _____   No: _____

I authorize the release of my STD/HIV/AIDS results whether negative or positive to the Above named person. Yes: _____   No: _____

I authorize the release of any record regarding drug, alcohol or mental treatment to the Above named person.

Patient Signature		Date Signed	

This authorization expires ninety days after it is issued.

Medical Release	
Patient's name	Date of Birth
Previous name	Social Security number
I request and authorize _____ to release healthcare information of The above named patient.	
Name	Address
City	State	Zip code

This request and authorization applies to _____

Healthcare information relating to the following condition, treatment and dates:
All healthcare information:
Other:
Yes: _____   No: _____

I authorize the release of my STD/HIV/AIDS results whether negative or positive to the Above named person. Yes: _____   No: _____

I authorize the release of any record regarding drug, alcohol or mental treatment to the Above named person.

Patient Signature		Date Signed	

This authorization expires ninety days after it is issued.

Medical Release

Patient's name	Date of Birth
Previous name	Social Security number

I request and authorize _____ to release healthcare information of
The above named patient.

Name	Address

City	State	Zip code

This request and authorization applies to _____

Healthcare information relating to the following condition, treatment and dates:
All healthcare information:
Other:
Yes: _____ No: _____

I authorize the release of my STD/HIV/AIDS results whether negative or positive to the
Above named person. Yes: _____ No: _____

I authorize the release of any record regarding drug, alcohol or mental treatment to the
Above named person.

Patient Signature		Date Signed	

This authorization expires ninety days after it is issued.

Medical Release	
Patient's name	Date of Birth
Previous name	Social Security number

I request and authorize _____ to release healthcare information of The above named patient.

Name	Address

City	State	Zip code

This request and authorization applies to _____

Healthcare information relating to the following condition, treatment and dates:
All healthcare information:
Other:
Yes: _____ No: _____

I authorize the release of my STD/HIV/AIDS results whether negative or positive to the
Above named person. Yes: _____ No: _____

I authorize the release of any record regarding drug, alcohol or mental treatment to the
Above named person.

Patient Signature		Date Signed	

This authorization expires ninety days after it is issued.

Medical Release	
Patient's name	Date of Birth
Previous name	Social Security number

I request and authorize _____ to release healthcare information of The above named patient.		
Name		Address
City	State	Zip code
This request and authorization applies to _____		
Healthcare information relating to the following condition, treatment and dates: All healthcare information: Other: Yes: _____ No: _____		
I authorize the release of my STD/HIV/AIDS results whether negative or positive to the Above named person. Yes: _____ No: _____		
I authorize the release of any record regarding drug, alcohol or mental treatment to the Above named person.		
Patient Signature		Date Signed	
This authorization expires ninety days after it is issued.			

Medical Release	
Patient's name	Date of Birth
Previous name	Social Security number

I request and authorize _____ to release healthcare information of The above named patient.

Name	Address

City	State	Zip code

This request and authorization applies to _____

Healthcare information relating to the following condition, treatment and dates:
All healthcare information:
Other:
Yes: _____ No: _____

I authorize the release of my STD/HIV/AIDS results whether negative or positive to the Above named person. Yes: _____ No: _____

I authorize the release of any record regarding drug, alcohol or mental treatment to the Above named person.

Patient Signature		Date Signed	

This authorization expires ninety days after it is issued.

Medical Release	
Patient's name	Date of Birth
Previous name	Social Security number

I request and authorize _____ to release healthcare information of
The above named patient.

Name	Address

City	State	Zip code

This request and authorization applies to _____

Healthcare information relating to the following condition, treatment and dates:
All healthcare information:
Other:
Yes: _____ No: _____

I authorize the release of my STD/HIV/AIDS results whether negative or positive to the
Above named person. Yes: _____ No: _____

I authorize the release of any record regarding drug, alcohol or mental treatment to the
Above named person.

Patient Signature		Date Signed	

This authorization expires ninety days after it is issued.

Medical Release

Patient's name	Date of Birth

Previous name	Social Security number

I request and authorize _____ to release healthcare information of
The above named patient.

Name	Address

City	State	Zip code

This request and authorization applies to _____

Healthcare information relating to the following condition, treatment and dates:
All healthcare information:
Other:
Yes: _____   No: _____

I authorize the release of my STD/HIV/AIDS results whether negative or positive to the
Above named person. Yes: _____   No: _____

I authorize the release of any record regarding drug, alcohol or mental treatment to the
Above named person.

Patient Signature		Date Signed	

This authorization expires ninety days after it is issued.

Medical Release

Patient's name	Date of Birth

Previous name	Social Security number

I request and authorize _____ to release healthcare information of
The above named patient.

Name	Address

City	State	Zip code

This request and authorization applies to _____

Healthcare information relating to the following condition, treatment and dates:
All healthcare information:
Other:
Yes: _____ No: _____

I authorize the release of my STD/HIV/AIDS results whether negative or positive to the
Above named person. Yes: _____ No: _____

I authorize the release of any record regarding drug, alcohol or mental treatment to the
Above named person.

Patient Signature		Date Signed	

This authorization expires ninety days after it is issued.

Medical Release	
Patient's name	Date of Birth
Previous name	Social Security number

I request and authorize _____ to release healthcare information of
The above named patient.

Name	Address

City	State	Zip code

This request and authorization applies to _____

Healthcare information relating to the following condition, treatment and dates:
All healthcare information:
Other:
Yes: _____ No: _____

I authorize the release of my STD/HIV/AIDS results whether negative or positive to the
Above named person. Yes: _____ No: _____

I authorize the release of any record regarding drug, alcohol or mental treatment to the
Above named person.

Patient Signature		Date Signed	

This authorization expires ninety days after it is issued.

Medical Release	
Patient's name	Date of Birth
Previous name	Social Security number
I request and authorize _____ to release healthcare information of The above named patient.	
Name	Address
City	State	Zip code

This request and authorization applies to _____
Healthcare information relating to the following condition, treatment and dates: All healthcare information: Other: Yes: _____ No: _____
I authorize the release of my STD/HIV/AIDS results whether negative or positive to the Above named person. Yes: _____ No: _____
I authorize the release of any record regarding drug, alcohol or mental treatment to the Above named person.

Patient Signature		Date Signed	
This authorization expires ninety days after it is issued.			

	Medical Release		
	Patient's name		Date of Birth
	Previous name		Social Security number

I request and authorize _____ to release healthcare information of
The above named patient.

Name	Address

City	State	Zip code

This request and authorization applies to _____

Healthcare information relating to the following condition, treatment and dates:
All healthcare information:
Other:
Yes: _____   No: _____

I authorize the release of my STD/HIV/AIDS results whether negative or positive to the
Above named person. Yes: _____   No: _____

I authorize the release of any record regarding drug, alcohol or mental treatment to the
Above named person.

Patient Signature		Date Signed	

This authorization expires ninety days after it is issued.

Medical Release	
Patient's name	Date of Birth
Previous name	Social Security number

I request and authorize _____ to release healthcare information of
The above named patient.

Name		Address	
City	State		Zip code

This request and authorization applies to _____

Healthcare information relating to the following condition, treatment and dates:
All healthcare information:
Other:
Yes: _____   No: _____

I authorize the release of my STD/HIV/AIDS results whether negative or positive to the
Above named person. Yes: _____   No: _____

I authorize the release of any record regarding drug, alcohol or mental treatment to the
Above named person.

Patient Signature		Date Signed	

This authorization expires ninety days after it is issued.

Medical Release

Patient's name	Date of Birth

Previous name	Social Security number

I request and authorize _____ to release healthcare information of
The above named patient.

Name	Address

City	State	Zip code

This request and authorization applies to _____

Healthcare information relating to the following condition, treatment and dates:
All healthcare information:
Other:
Yes: _____ No: _____

I authorize the release of my STD/HIV/AIDS results whether negative or positive to the
Above named person. Yes: _____ No: _____

I authorize the release of any record regarding drug, alcohol or mental treatment to the
Above named person.

Patient Signature		Date Signed	

This authorization expires ninety days after it is issued.

Medical Release	
Patient's name	Date of Birth
Previous name	Social Security number

I request and authorize _____ to release healthcare information of The above named patient.			
Name			Address
City	State		Zip code
This request and authorization applies to _____			
Healthcare information relating to the following condition, treatment and dates: All healthcare information: Other: Yes: _____ No: _____			
I authorize the release of my STD/HIV/AIDS results whether negative or positive to the Above named person. Yes: _____ No: _____			
I authorize the release of any record regarding drug, alcohol or mental treatment to the Above named person.			
Patient Signature		Date Signed	
This authorization expires ninety days after it is issued.			

Medical Release	
Patient's name	Date of Birth
Previous name	Social Security number
I request and authorize _____ to release healthcare information of The above named patient.	
Name	Address
City	State	Zip code
This request and authorization applies to _____	
Healthcare information relating to the following condition, treatment and dates: All healthcare information: Other: Yes: _____ No: _____	
I authorize the release of my STD/HIV/AIDS results whether negative or positive to the Above named person. Yes: _____ No: _____	
I authorize the release of any record regarding drug, alcohol or mental treatment to the Above named person.	
Patient Signature		Date Signed	
This authorization expires ninety days after it is issued.	

Medical Release	
Patient's name	Date of Birth
Previous name	Social Security number

I request and authorize _____ to release healthcare information of The above named patient.

Name	Address

City	State	Zip code

This request and authorization applies to _____
Healthcare information relating to the following condition, treatment and dates: All healthcare information: Other: Yes: _____ No: _____
I authorize the release of my STD/HIV/AIDS results whether negative or positive to the Above named person. Yes: _____ No: _____
I authorize the release of any record regarding drug, alcohol or mental treatment to the Above named person.

Patient Signature		Date Signed	

This authorization expires ninety days after it is issued.

Medical Release

Patient's name	Date of Birth

Previous name	Social Security number

I request and authorize _____ to release healthcare information of
The above named patient.

Name	Address

City	State	Zip code

This request and authorization applies to _____

Healthcare information relating to the following condition, treatment and dates:
All healthcare information:
Other:
Yes: _____   No: _____

I authorize the release of my STD/HIV/AIDS results whether negative or positive to the
Above named person. Yes: _____   No: _____

I authorize the release of any record regarding drug, alcohol or mental treatment to the
Above named person.

Patient Signature		Date Signed	

This authorization expires ninety days after it is issued.

Medical Release	
Patient's name	Date of Birth
Previous name	Social Security number

I request and authorize _____ to release healthcare information of
The above named patient.

Name	Address

City	State	Zip code

This request and authorization applies to _____

Healthcare information relating to the following condition, treatment and dates:
All healthcare information:
Other:
Yes: _____ No: _____

I authorize the release of my STD/HIV/AIDS results whether negative or positive to the
Above named person. Yes: _____ No: _____

I authorize the release of any record regarding drug, alcohol or mental treatment to the
Above named person.

Patient Signature		Date Signed	

This authorization expires ninety days after it is issued.

Medical Release	
Patient's name	Date of Birth
Previous name	Social Security number
I request and authorize _____ to release healthcare information of The above named patient.	
Name	Address

City	State	Zip code

This request and authorization applies to _____

Healthcare information relating to the following condition, treatment and dates:
All healthcare information:
Other:
Yes: _____   No: _____

I authorize the release of my STD/HIV/AIDS results whether negative or positive to the Above named person. Yes: _____   No: _____

I authorize the release of any record regarding drug, alcohol or mental treatment to the Above named person.

Patient Signature		Date Signed	

This authorization expires ninety days after it is issued.

Medical Release	
Patient's name	Date of Birth
Previous name	Social Security number

I request and authorize _____ to release healthcare information of
The above named patient.

Name	Address

City	State	Zip code

This request and authorization applies to _____

Healthcare information relating to the following condition, treatment and dates:
All healthcare information:
Other:
Yes: _____ No: _____

I authorize the release of my STD/HIV/AIDS results whether negative or positive to the
Above named person. Yes: _____ No: _____

I authorize the release of any record regarding drug, alcohol or mental treatment to the
Above named person.

Patient Signature		Date Signed	

This authorization expires ninety days after it is issued.

Medical Release	
Patient's name	Date of Birth
Previous name	Social Security number

I request and authorize _____ to release healthcare information of The above named patient.

Name	Address

City	State	Zip code

This request and authorization applies to _____

Healthcare information relating to the following condition, treatment and dates:
All healthcare information:
Other:
Yes: _____ No: _____

I authorize the release of my STD/HIV/AIDS results whether negative or positive to the Above named person. Yes: _____ No: _____

I authorize the release of any record regarding drug, alcohol or mental treatment to the Above named person.

Patient Signature		Date Signed	

This authorization expires ninety days after it is issued.

Medical Release

Patient's name	Date of Birth

Previous name	Social Security number

I request and authorize _____ to release healthcare information of The above named patient.

Name	Address

City	State	Zip code

This request and authorization applies to _____

Healthcare information relating to the following condition, treatment and dates:
All healthcare information:
Other:
Yes: _____ No: _____

I authorize the release of my STD/HIV/AIDS results whether negative or positive to the Above named person. Yes: _____ No: _____

I authorize the release of any record regarding drug, alcohol or mental treatment to the Above named person.

Patient Signature		Date Signed	

This authorization expires ninety days after it is issued.

Medical Release	
Patient's name	Date of Birth
Previous name	Social Security number

I request and authorize _____ to release healthcare information of
The above named patient.

Name	Address

City	State	Zip code

This request and authorization applies to _____

Healthcare information relating to the following condition, treatment and dates:
All healthcare information:
Other:
Yes: _____   No: _____

I authorize the release of my STD/HIV/AIDS results whether negative or positive to the
Above named person. Yes: _____   No: _____

I authorize the release of any record regarding drug, alcohol or mental treatment to the
Above named person.

Patient Signature		Date Signed	

This authorization expires ninety days after it is issued.

Medical Release	
Patient's name	Date of Birth
Previous name	Social Security number

I request and authorize _____ to release healthcare information of The above named patient.

Name	Address

City	State	Zip code

This request and authorization applies to _____

Healthcare information relating to the following condition, treatment and dates:
All healthcare information:
Other:
Yes: _____ No: _____

I authorize the release of my STD/HIV/AIDS results whether negative or positive to the Above named person. Yes: _____ No: _____

I authorize the release of any record regarding drug, alcohol or mental treatment to the Above named person.

Patient Signature		Date Signed	

This authorization expires ninety days after it is issued.

Medical Release	
Patient's name	Date of Birth
Previous name	Social Security number

I request and authorize _____ to release healthcare information of
The above named patient.

Name	Address

City	State	Zip code

This request and authorization applies to _____

Healthcare information relating to the following condition, treatment and dates:
All healthcare information:
Other:
Yes: _____ No: _____

I authorize the release of my STD/HIV/AIDS results whether negative or positive to the
Above named person. Yes: _____ No: _____

I authorize the release of any record regarding drug, alcohol or mental treatment to the
Above named person.

Patient Signature		Date Signed	

This authorization expires ninety days after it is issued.

	Medical Release	
Patient's name		Date of Birth
Previous name		Social Security number

I request and authorize _____ to release healthcare information of
The above named patient.

Name	Address

City	State	Zip code

This request and authorization applies to _____

Healthcare information relating to the following condition, treatment and dates:
All healthcare information:
Other:
Yes: _____   No: _____

I authorize the release of my STD/HIV/AIDS results whether negative or positive to the
Above named person. Yes: _____   No: _____

I authorize the release of any record regarding drug, alcohol or mental treatment to the
Above named person.

Patient Signature		Date Signed	

This authorization expires ninety days after it is issued.

Medical Release	
Patient's name	Date of Birth
Previous name	Social Security number

I request and authorize _____ to release healthcare information of The above named patient.		
Name		Address
City	State	Zip code
This request and authorization applies to _____		
Healthcare information relating to the following condition, treatment and dates: All healthcare information: Other: Yes: _____ No: _____		
I authorize the release of my STD/HIV/AIDS results whether negative or positive to the Above named person. Yes: _____ No: _____		
I authorize the release of any record regarding drug, alcohol or mental treatment to the Above named person.		
Patient Signature		Date Signed	
This authorization expires ninety days after it is issued.			

Medical Release	
Patient's name	Date of Birth
Previous name	Social Security number

I request and authorize _____ to release healthcare information of The above named patient.			
Name			Address
City	State		Zip code
This request and authorization applies to _____			
Healthcare information relating to the following condition, treatment and dates: All healthcare information: Other: Yes: _____ No: _____			
I authorize the release of my STD/HIV/AIDS results whether negative or positive to the Above named person. Yes: _____ No: _____			
I authorize the release of any record regarding drug, alcohol or mental treatment to the Above named person.			
Patient Signature		Date Signed	
This authorization expires ninety days after it is issued.			

Medical Release	
Patient's name	Date of Birth
Previous name	Social Security number

I request and authorize _____ to release healthcare information of The above named patient.

Name	Address

City	State	Zip code

This request and authorization applies to _____

Healthcare information relating to the following condition, treatment and dates:
All healthcare information:
Other:
Yes: _____ No: _____

I authorize the release of my STD/HIV/AIDS results whether negative or positive to the Above named person. Yes: _____ No: _____

I authorize the release of any record regarding drug, alcohol or mental treatment to the Above named person.

Patient Signature		Date Signed	

This authorization expires ninety days after it is issued.

Medical Release	
Patient's name	Date of Birth
Previous name	Social Security number
I request and authorize _____ to release healthcare information of The above named patient.	
Name	Address

City	State	Zip code

This request and authorization applies to _____

Healthcare information relating to the following condition, treatment and dates:
All healthcare information:
Other:
Yes: _____ No: _____

I authorize the release of my STD/HIV/AIDS results whether negative or positive to the
Above named person. Yes: _____ No: _____

I authorize the release of any record regarding drug, alcohol or mental treatment to the
Above named person.

Patient Signature		Date Signed	

This authorization expires ninety days after it is issued.

Medical Release

Patient's name	Date of Birth

Previous name	Social Security number

I request and authorize _____ to release healthcare information of
The above named patient.

Name	Address

City	State	Zip code

This request and authorization applies to _____

Healthcare information relating to the following condition, treatment and dates:
All healthcare information:
Other:
Yes: _____ No: _____

I authorize the release of my STD/HIV/AIDS results whether negative or positive to the
Above named person. Yes: _____ No: _____

I authorize the release of any record regarding drug, alcohol or mental treatment to the
Above named person.

Patient Signature		Date Signed	

This authorization expires ninety days after it is issued.

Medical Release	
Patient's name	Date of Birth
Previous name	Social Security number

I request and authorize _____ to release healthcare information of The above named patient.		
Name		Address
City	State	Zip code
This request and authorization applies to _____		
Healthcare information relating to the following condition, treatment and dates: All healthcare information: Other: Yes: _____ No: _____		
I authorize the release of my STD/HIV/AIDS results whether negative or positive to the Above named person. Yes: _____ No: _____		
I authorize the release of any record regarding drug, alcohol or mental treatment to the Above named person.		
Patient Signature		Date Signed	
This authorization expires ninety days after it is issued.		

Medical Release

Patient's name	Date of Birth

Previous name	Social Security number

I request and authorize _____ to release healthcare information of
The above named patient.

Name	Address

City	State	Zip code

This request and authorization applies to _____

Healthcare information relating to the following condition, treatment and dates:
All healthcare information:
Other:
Yes: _____   No: _____

I authorize the release of my STD/HIV/AIDS results whether negative or positive to the Above named person. Yes: _____   No: _____

I authorize the release of any record regarding drug, alcohol or mental treatment to the Above named person.

Patient Signature		Date Signed	

This authorization expires ninety days after it is issued.

<div align="center">**Medical Release**</div>	
<div align="center">Patient's name</div>	<div align="center">Date of Birth</div>
<div align="center">Previous name</div>	<div align="center">Social Security number</div>

I request and authorize _____ to release healthcare information of
The above named patient.

Name	Address

City	State	Zip code

This request and authorization applies to _____

Healthcare information relating to the following condition, treatment and dates:
All healthcare information:
Other:
Yes: _____   No: _____

I authorize the release of my STD/HIV/AIDS results whether negative or positive to the
Above named person. Yes: _____   No: _____

I authorize the release of any record regarding drug, alcohol or mental treatment to the
Above named person.

Patient Signature		Date Signed	

This authorization expires ninety days after it is issued.

Medical Release	
Patient's name	Date of Birth
Previous name	Social Security number

I request and authorize _____ to release healthcare information of The above named patient.		
Name		Address
City	State	Zip code
This request and authorization applies to _____		
Healthcare information relating to the following condition, treatment and dates: All healthcare information: Other: Yes: _____ No: _____		
I authorize the release of my STD/HIV/AIDS results whether negative or positive to the Above named person. Yes: _____ No: _____		
I authorize the release of any record regarding drug, alcohol or mental treatment to the Above named person.		
Patient Signature		Date Signed	
This authorization expires ninety days after it is issued.		

Medical Release	
Patient's name	Date of Birth
Previous name	Social Security number

I request and authorize _____ to release healthcare information of
The above named patient.

Name	Address

City	State	Zip code

This request and authorization applies to _____

Healthcare information relating to the following condition, treatment and dates:
All healthcare information:
Other:
Yes: _____   No: _____

I authorize the release of my STD/HIV/AIDS results whether negative or positive to the
Above named person. Yes: _____   No: _____

I authorize the release of any record regarding drug, alcohol or mental treatment to the
Above named person.

Patient Signature		Date Signed	

This authorization expires ninety days after it is issued.

Medical Release	
Patient's name	Date of Birth
Previous name	Social Security number

I request and authorize _____ to release healthcare information of
The above named patient.

Name	Address

City	State	Zip code

This request and authorization applies to _____

Healthcare information relating to the following condition, treatment and dates:
All healthcare information:
Other:
Yes: _____ No: _____

I authorize the release of my STD/HIV/AIDS results whether negative or positive to the
Above named person. Yes: _____ No: _____

I authorize the release of any record regarding drug, alcohol or mental treatment to the
Above named person.

Patient Signature		Date Signed	

This authorization expires ninety days after it is issued.

Medical Release

Patient's name	Date of Birth

Previous name	Social Security number

I request and authorize _____ to release healthcare information of
The above named patient.

Name	Address

City	State	Zip code

This request and authorization applies to _____

Healthcare information relating to the following condition, treatment and dates:
All healthcare information:
Other:
Yes: _____ No: _____

I authorize the release of my STD/HIV/AIDS results whether negative or positive to the
Above named person. Yes: _____ No: _____

I authorize the release of any record regarding drug, alcohol or mental treatment to the
Above named person.

Patient Signature		Date Signed	

This authorization expires ninety days after it is issued.

Medical Release	
Patient's name	Date of Birth
Previous name	Social Security number
I request and authorize _____ to release healthcare information of The above named patient.	
Name	Address

City	State	Zip code

This request and authorization applies to _____

Healthcare information relating to the following condition, treatment and dates:
All healthcare information:
Other:
Yes: _____ No: _____

I authorize the release of my STD/HIV/AIDS results whether negative or positive to the
Above named person. Yes: _____ No: _____

I authorize the release of any record regarding drug, alcohol or mental treatment to the
Above named person.

Patient Signature		Date Signed	

This authorization expires ninety days after it is issued.

Patient's name	Date of Birth
Previous name	Social Security number

I request and authorize _____ to release healthcare information of The above named patient.

Name	Address

City	State	Zip code

This request and authorization applies to _____

Healthcare information relating to the following condition, treatment and dates:
All healthcare information:
Other:
Yes: _____   No: _____

I authorize the release of my STD/HIV/AIDS results whether negative or positive to the Above named person. Yes: _____   No: _____

I authorize the release of any record regarding drug, alcohol or mental treatment to the Above named person.

Patient Signature		Date Signed	

This authorization expires ninety days after it is issued.

Medical Release	
Patient's name	Date of Birth
Previous name	Social Security number

I request and authorize _____ to release healthcare information of
The above named patient.

Name	Address

City	State	Zip code

This request and authorization applies to _____

Healthcare information relating to the following condition, treatment and dates:
All healthcare information:
Other:
Yes: _____ No: _____

I authorize the release of my STD/HIV/AIDS results whether negative or positive to the
Above named person. Yes: _____ No: _____

I authorize the release of any record regarding drug, alcohol or mental treatment to the
Above named person.

Patient Signature		Date Signed	

This authorization expires ninety days after it is issued.

Medical Release	
Patient's name	Date of Birth
Previous name	Social Security number

I request and authorize _____ to release healthcare information of The above named patient.			
Name		Address	
City	State		Zip code
This request and authorization applies to _____			
Healthcare information relating to the following condition, treatment and dates: All healthcare information: Other: Yes: _____ No: _____			
I authorize the release of my STD/HIV/AIDS results whether negative or positive to the Above named person. Yes: _____ No: _____			
I authorize the release of any record regarding drug, alcohol or mental treatment to the Above named person.			
Patient Signature		Date Signed	
This authorization expires ninety days after it is issued.			

Medical Release	
Patient's name	Date of Birth
Previous name	Social Security number

I request and authorize _____ to release healthcare information of
The above named patient.

Name	Address

City	State	Zip code

This request and authorization applies to _____

Healthcare information relating to the following condition, treatment and dates:
All healthcare information:
Other:
Yes: _____ No: _____

I authorize the release of my STD/HIV/AIDS results whether negative or positive to the
Above named person. Yes: _____ No: _____

I authorize the release of any record regarding drug, alcohol or mental treatment to the
Above named person.

Patient Signature		Date Signed	

This authorization expires ninety days after it is issued.

Medical Release

Patient's name	Date of Birth

Previous name	Social Security number

I request and authorize _____ to release healthcare information of The above named patient.

Name	Address

City	State	Zip code

This request and authorization applies to _____

Healthcare information relating to the following condition, treatment and dates:
All healthcare information:
Other:
Yes: _____ No: _____

I authorize the release of my STD/HIV/AIDS results whether negative or positive to the Above named person. Yes: _____ No: _____

I authorize the release of any record regarding drug, alcohol or mental treatment to the Above named person.

Patient Signature		Date Signed	

This authorization expires ninety days after it is issued.

Medical Release

Patient's name	Date of Birth

Previous name	Social Security number

I request and authorize _____ to release healthcare information of
The above named patient.

Name	Address

City	State	Zip code

This request and authorization applies to _____

Healthcare information relating to the following condition, treatment and dates:
All healthcare information:
Other:
Yes: _____ No: _____

I authorize the release of my STD/HIV/AIDS results whether negative or positive to the
Above named person. Yes: _____ No: _____

I authorize the release of any record regarding drug, alcohol or mental treatment to the
Above named person.

Patient Signature		Date Signed	

This authorization expires ninety days after it is issued.

Medical Release

Patient's name	Date of Birth
Previous name	Social Security number

I request and authorize _____ to release healthcare information of
The above named patient.

Name	Address

City	State	Zip code

This request and authorization applies to _____

Healthcare information relating to the following condition, treatment and dates:
All healthcare information:
Other:
Yes: _____   No: _____

I authorize the release of my STD/HIV/AIDS results whether negative or positive to the
Above named person. Yes: _____   No: _____

I authorize the release of any record regarding drug, alcohol or mental treatment to the
Above named person.

Patient Signature		Date Signed	

This authorization expires ninety days after it is issued.

Medical Release	
Patient's name	Date of Birth
Previous name	Social Security number

I request and authorize _____ to release healthcare information of The above named patient.

Name	Address

City	State	Zip code

This request and authorization applies to _____

Healthcare information relating to the following condition, treatment and dates:
All healthcare information:
Other:
Yes: _____   No: _____

I authorize the release of my STD/HIV/AIDS results whether negative or positive to the Above named person. Yes: _____   No: _____

I authorize the release of any record regarding drug, alcohol or mental treatment to the Above named person.

Patient Signature		Date Signed	

This authorization expires ninety days after it is issued.

Medical Release

Patient's name	Date of Birth

Previous name	Social Security number

I request and authorize _____ to release healthcare information of
The above named patient.

Name	Address

City	State	Zip code

This request and authorization applies to _____

Healthcare information relating to the following condition, treatment and dates:
All healthcare information:
Other:
Yes: _____   No: _____

I authorize the release of my STD/HIV/AIDS results whether negative or positive to the
Above named person. Yes: _____   No: _____

I authorize the release of any record regarding drug, alcohol or mental treatment to the
Above named person.

Patient Signature		Date Signed	

This authorization expires ninety days after it is issued.

Medical Release

Patient's name	Date of Birth

Previous name	Social Security number

I request and authorize _____ to release healthcare information of
The above named patient.

Name	Address

City	State	Zip code

This request and authorization applies to _____

Healthcare information relating to the following condition, treatment and dates:
All healthcare information:
Other:
Yes: _____ No: _____

I authorize the release of my STD/HIV/AIDS results whether negative or positive to the
Above named person. Yes: _____ No: _____

I authorize the release of any record regarding drug, alcohol or mental treatment to the
Above named person.

Patient Signature		Date Signed	

This authorization expires ninety days after it is issued.

Medical Release	
Patient's name	Date of Birth
Previous name	Social Security number

I request and authorize _____ to release healthcare information of
The above named patient.

Name	Address

City	State	Zip code

This request and authorization applies to _____

Healthcare information relating to the following condition, treatment and dates:
All healthcare information:
Other:
Yes: _____ No: _____

I authorize the release of my STD/HIV/AIDS results whether negative or positive to the
Above named person. Yes: _____ No: _____

I authorize the release of any record regarding drug, alcohol or mental treatment to the
Above named person.

Patient Signature		Date Signed	

This authorization expires ninety days after it is issued.

Medical Release	
Patient's name	Date of Birth
Previous name	Social Security number

I request and authorize _____ to release healthcare information of The above named patient.			
Name		Address	
City	State		Zip code
This request and authorization applies to _____			
Healthcare information relating to the following condition, treatment and dates: All healthcare information: Other: Yes: _____ No: _____			
I authorize the release of my STD/HIV/AIDS results whether negative or positive to the Above named person. Yes: _____ No: _____			
I authorize the release of any record regarding drug, alcohol or mental treatment to the Above named person.			
Patient Signature		Date Signed	
This authorization expires ninety days after it is issued.			

Medical Release	
Patient's name	Date of Birth
Previous name	Social Security number

I request and authorize _____ to release healthcare information of
The above named patient.

Name	Address

City	State	Zip code

This request and authorization applies to _____

Healthcare information relating to the following condition, treatment and dates:
All healthcare information:
Other:
Yes: _____ No: _____

I authorize the release of my STD/HIV/AIDS results whether negative or positive to the
Above named person. Yes: _____ No: _____

I authorize the release of any record regarding drug, alcohol or mental treatment to the
Above named person.

Patient Signature		Date Signed	

This authorization expires ninety days after it is issued.

Medical Release	
Patient's name	Date of Birth
Previous name	Social Security number

I request and authorize _____ to release healthcare information of
The above named patient.

Name	Address

City	State	Zip code

This request and authorization applies to _____

Healthcare information relating to the following condition, treatment and dates:
All healthcare information:
Other:
Yes: _____ No: _____

I authorize the release of my STD/HIV/AIDS results whether negative or positive to the
Above named person. Yes: _____ No: _____

I authorize the release of any record regarding drug, alcohol or mental treatment to the
Above named person.

Patient Signature		Date Signed	

This authorization expires ninety days after it is issued.

Medical Release

Patient's name	Date of Birth

Previous name	Social Security number

I request and authorize _____ to release healthcare information of
The above named patient.

Name	Address

City	State	Zip code

This request and authorization applies to _____

Healthcare information relating to the following condition, treatment and dates:
All healthcare information:
Other:
Yes: _____ No: _____

I authorize the release of my STD/HIV/AIDS results whether negative or positive to the
Above named person. Yes: _____ No: _____

I authorize the release of any record regarding drug, alcohol or mental treatment to the
Above named person.

Patient Signature		Date Signed	

This authorization expires ninety days after it is issued.

Medical Release	
Patient's name	Date of Birth
Previous name	Social Security number

I request and authorize _____ to release healthcare information of The above named patient.		
Name		Address
City	State	Zip code
This request and authorization applies to _____		
Healthcare information relating to the following condition, treatment and dates: All healthcare information: Other: Yes: _____ No: _____		
I authorize the release of my STD/HIV/AIDS results whether negative or positive to the Above named person. Yes: _____ No: _____		
I authorize the release of any record regarding drug, alcohol or mental treatment to the Above named person.		
Patient Signature		Date Signed	
This authorization expires ninety days after it is issued.			

Medical Release	
Patient's name	Date of Birth
Previous name	Social Security number

I request and authorize _____ to release healthcare information of The above named patient.		
Name		Address
City	State	Zip code
This request and authorization applies to _____		
Healthcare information relating to the following condition, treatment and dates: All healthcare information: Other: Yes: _____ No: _____		
I authorize the release of my STD/HIV/AIDS results whether negative or positive to the Above named person. Yes: _____ No: _____		
I authorize the release of any record regarding drug, alcohol or mental treatment to the Above named person.		
Patient Signature		Date Signed
This authorization expires ninety days after it is issued.		

Medical Release

Patient's name	Date of Birth
Previous name	Social Security number

I request and authorize _____ to release healthcare information of The above named patient.

Name	Address

City	State	Zip code

This request and authorization applies to _____

Healthcare information relating to the following condition, treatment and dates:
All healthcare information:
Other:
Yes: _____ No: _____

I authorize the release of my STD/HIV/AIDS results whether negative or positive to the Above named person. Yes: _____ No: _____

I authorize the release of any record regarding drug, alcohol or mental treatment to the Above named person.

Patient Signature		Date Signed	

This authorization expires ninety days after it is issued.

Medical Release

Patient's name	Date of Birth

Previous name	Social Security number

I request and authorize _____ to release healthcare information of
The above named patient.

Name	Address

City	State	Zip code

This request and authorization applies to _____

Healthcare information relating to the following condition, treatment and dates:
All healthcare information:
Other:
Yes: _____ No: _____

I authorize the release of my STD/HIV/AIDS results whether negative or positive to the
Above named person. Yes: _____ No: _____

I authorize the release of any record regarding drug, alcohol or mental treatment to the
Above named person.

Patient Signature		Date Signed	

This authorization expires ninety days after it is issued.

Medical Release	
Patient's name	Date of Birth
Previous name	Social Security number

I request and authorize _____ to release healthcare information of The above named patient.		
Name		Address
City	State	Zip code
This request and authorization applies to _____		
Healthcare information relating to the following condition, treatment and dates: All healthcare information: Other: Yes: _____ No: _____		
I authorize the release of my STD/HIV/AIDS results whether negative or positive to the Above named person. Yes: _____ No: _____		
I authorize the release of any record regarding drug, alcohol or mental treatment to the Above named person.		
Patient Signature		Date Signed	
This authorization expires ninety days after it is issued.			

Medical Release

Patient's name	Date of Birth

Previous name	Social Security number

I request and authorize _____ to release healthcare information of
The above named patient.

Name	Address

City	State	Zip code

This request and authorization applies to _____

Healthcare information relating to the following condition, treatment and dates:
All healthcare information:
Other:
Yes: _____   No: _____

I authorize the release of my STD/HIV/AIDS results whether negative or positive to the Above named person. Yes: _____   No: _____

I authorize the release of any record regarding drug, alcohol or mental treatment to the Above named person.

Patient Signature		Date Signed	

This authorization expires ninety days after it is issued.

Medical Release

Patient's name	Date of Birth

Previous name	Social Security number

I request and authorize _____ to release healthcare information of
The above named patient.

Name	Address

City	State	Zip code

This request and authorization applies to _____

Healthcare information relating to the following condition, treatment and dates:
All healthcare information:
Other:
Yes: _____   No: _____

I authorize the release of my STD/HIV/AIDS results whether negative or positive to the
Above named person. Yes: _____   No: _____

I authorize the release of any record regarding drug, alcohol or mental treatment to the
Above named person.

Patient Signature		Date Signed	

This authorization expires ninety days after it is issued.

Medical Release	
Patient's name	Date of Birth
Previous name	Social Security number

I request and authorize _____ to release healthcare information of The above named patient.			
Name		Address	
City	State		Zip code
This request and authorization applies to _____			
Healthcare information relating to the following condition, treatment and dates: All healthcare information: Other: Yes: _____ No: _____			
I authorize the release of my STD/HIV/AIDS results whether negative or positive to the Above named person. Yes: _____ No: _____			
I authorize the release of any record regarding drug, alcohol or mental treatment to the Above named person.			
Patient Signature		Date Signed	
This authorization expires ninety days after it is issued.			

Medical Release	
Patient's name	Date of Birth
Previous name	Social Security number

I request and authorize _____ to release healthcare information of The above named patient.	
Name	Address

City	State	Zip code

This request and authorization applies to _____

Healthcare information relating to the following condition, treatment and dates:
All healthcare information:
Other:
Yes: _____   No: _____

I authorize the release of my STD/HIV/AIDS results whether negative or positive to the Above named person. Yes: _____   No: _____

I authorize the release of any record regarding drug, alcohol or mental treatment to the Above named person.

Patient Signature		Date Signed	

This authorization expires ninety days after it is issued.

Medical Release	
Patient's name	Date of Birth
Previous name	Social Security number

I request and authorize _____ to release healthcare information of
The above named patient.

Name	Address

City	State	Zip code

This request and authorization applies to _____

Healthcare information relating to the following condition, treatment and dates:
All healthcare information:
Other:
Yes: _____ No: _____

I authorize the release of my STD/HIV/AIDS results whether negative or positive to the
Above named person. Yes: _____ No: _____

I authorize the release of any record regarding drug, alcohol or mental treatment to the
Above named person.

Patient Signature		Date Signed	

This authorization expires ninety days after it is issued.

Medical Release	
Patient's name	Date of Birth
Previous name	Social Security number

I request and authorize _____ to release healthcare information of
The above named patient.

Name	Address

City	State	Zip code

This request and authorization applies to _____

Healthcare information relating to the following condition, treatment and dates:
All healthcare information:
Other:
Yes: _____ No: _____

I authorize the release of my STD/HIV/AIDS results whether negative or positive to the
Above named person. Yes: _____ No: _____

I authorize the release of any record regarding drug, alcohol or mental treatment to the
Above named person.

Patient Signature		Date Signed	

This authorization expires ninety days after it is issued.

Medical Release	
Patient's name	Date of Birth
Previous name	Social Security number

I request and authorize _____ to release healthcare information of The above named patient.		
Name		Address
City	State	Zip code
This request and authorization applies to _____		
Healthcare information relating to the following condition, treatment and dates: All healthcare information: Other: Yes: _____ No: _____		
I authorize the release of my STD/HIV/AIDS results whether negative or positive to the Above named person. Yes: _____ No: _____		
I authorize the release of any record regarding drug, alcohol or mental treatment to the Above named person.		
Patient Signature		Date Signed	
This authorization expires ninety days after it is issued.		

Medical Release	
Patient's name	Date of Birth
Previous name	Social Security number

I request and authorize _____ to release healthcare information of The above named patient.

Name	Address

City	State	Zip code

This request and authorization applies to _____

Healthcare information relating to the following condition, treatment and dates:
All healthcare information:
Other:
Yes: _____   No: _____

I authorize the release of my STD/HIV/AIDS results whether negative or positive to the Above named person. Yes: _____   No: _____

I authorize the release of any record regarding drug, alcohol or mental treatment to the Above named person.

Patient Signature		Date Signed	

This authorization expires ninety days after it is issued.

Medical Release	
Patient's name	Date of Birth
Previous name	Social Security number

I request and authorize _____ to release healthcare information of The above named patient.

Name	Address

City	State	Zip code

This request and authorization applies to _____

Healthcare information relating to the following condition, treatment and dates:
All healthcare information:
Other:
Yes: _____ No: _____

I authorize the release of my STD/HIV/AIDS results whether negative or positive to the
Above named person. Yes: _____ No: _____

I authorize the release of any record regarding drug, alcohol or mental treatment to the
Above named person.

Patient Signature		Date Signed	

This authorization expires ninety days after it is issued.

Medical Release

Patient's name	Date of Birth

Previous name	Social Security number

I request and authorize _____ to release healthcare information of
The above named patient.

Name	Address

City	State	Zip code

This request and authorization applies to _____

Healthcare information relating to the following condition, treatment and dates:
All healthcare information:
Other:
Yes: _____ No: _____

I authorize the release of my STD/HIV/AIDS results whether negative or positive to the
Above named person. Yes: _____ No: _____

I authorize the release of any record regarding drug, alcohol or mental treatment to the
Above named person.

Patient Signature		Date Signed	

This authorization expires ninety days after it is issued.

Medical Release

Patient's name	Date of Birth

Previous name	Social Security number

I request and authorize _____ to release healthcare information of The above named patient.

Name	Address

City	State	Zip code

This request and authorization applies to _____

Healthcare information relating to the following condition, treatment and dates:
All healthcare information:
Other:
Yes: _____ No: _____

I authorize the release of my STD/HIV/AIDS results whether negative or positive to the Above named person. Yes: _____ No: _____

I authorize the release of any record regarding drug, alcohol or mental treatment to the Above named person.

Patient Signature		Date Signed	

This authorization expires ninety days after it is issued.

Medical Release	
Patient's name	Date of Birth
Previous name	Social Security number

I request and authorize _____ to release healthcare information of
The above named patient.

Name	Address

City	State	Zip code

This request and authorization applies to _____

Healthcare information relating to the following condition, treatment and dates:
All healthcare information:
Other:
Yes: _____ No: _____

I authorize the release of my STD/HIV/AIDS results whether negative or positive to the
Above named person. Yes: _____ No: _____

I authorize the release of any record regarding drug, alcohol or mental treatment to the
Above named person.

Patient Signature		Date Signed	

This authorization expires ninety days after it is issued.

Medical Release	
Patient's name	Date of Birth
Previous name	Social Security number
I request and authorize _____ to release healthcare information of The above named patient.	
Name	Address

City	State	Zip code

This request and authorization applies to _____
Healthcare information relating to the following condition, treatment and dates: All healthcare information: Other: Yes: _____ No: _____
I authorize the release of my STD/HIV/AIDS results whether negative or positive to the Above named person. Yes: _____ No: _____
I authorize the release of any record regarding drug, alcohol or mental treatment to the Above named person.

Patient Signature		Date Signed	
This authorization expires ninety days after it is issued.			

Medical Release

Patient's name	Date of Birth

Previous name	Social Security number

I request and authorize _____ to release healthcare information of
The above named patient.

Name	Address

City	State	Zip code

This request and authorization applies to _____

Healthcare information relating to the following condition, treatment and dates:
All healthcare information:
Other:
Yes: _____ No: _____

I authorize the release of my STD/HIV/AIDS results whether negative or positive to the Above named person. Yes: _____ No: _____

I authorize the release of any record regarding drug, alcohol or mental treatment to the Above named person.

Patient Signature		Date Signed	

This authorization expires ninety days after it is issued.

Medical Release	
Patient's name	Date of Birth
Previous name	Social Security number

I request and authorize _____ to release healthcare information of
The above named patient.

Name	Address

City	State	Zip code

This request and authorization applies to _____

Healthcare information relating to the following condition, treatment and dates:
All healthcare information:
Other:
Yes: _____ No: _____

I authorize the release of my STD/HIV/AIDS results whether negative or positive to the
Above named person. Yes: _____ No: _____

I authorize the release of any record regarding drug, alcohol or mental treatment to the
Above named person.

Patient Signature		Date Signed	

This authorization expires ninety days after it is issued.

Medical Release	
Patient's name	Date of Birth
Previous name	Social Security number

I request and authorize _____ to release healthcare information of The above named patient.			
Name		Address	
City	State		Zip code
This request and authorization applies to _____			
Healthcare information relating to the following condition, treatment and dates: All healthcare information: Other: Yes: _____ No: _____			
I authorize the release of my STD/HIV/AIDS results whether negative or positive to the Above named person. Yes: _____ No: _____			
I authorize the release of any record regarding drug, alcohol or mental treatment to the Above named person.			
Patient Signature		Date Signed	
This authorization expires ninety days after it is issued.			

Medical Release

Patient's name	Date of Birth

Previous name	Social Security number

I request and authorize _____ to release healthcare information of The above named patient.

Name	Address

City	State	Zip code

This request and authorization applies to _____

Healthcare information relating to the following condition, treatment and dates:
All healthcare information:
Other:
Yes: _____ No: _____

I authorize the release of my STD/HIV/AIDS results whether negative or positive to the Above named person. Yes: _____ No: _____

I authorize the release of any record regarding drug, alcohol or mental treatment to the Above named person.

Patient Signature		Date Signed	

This authorization expires ninety days after it is issued.

Medical Release	
Patient's name	Date of Birth
Previous name	Social Security number
I request and authorize _____ to release healthcare information of The above named patient.	
Name	Address
City	State	Zip code
This request and authorization applies to _____	
Healthcare information relating to the following condition, treatment and dates: All healthcare information: Other: Yes: _____ No: _____	
I authorize the release of my STD/HIV/AIDS results whether negative or positive to the Above named person. Yes: _____ No: _____	
I authorize the release of any record regarding drug, alcohol or mental treatment to the Above named person.	
Patient Signature		Date Signed	
This authorization expires ninety days after it is issued.	

Medical Release

Patient's name	Date of Birth

Previous name	Social Security number

I request and authorize _____ to release healthcare information of
The above named patient.

Name	Address

City	State	Zip code

This request and authorization applies to _____

Healthcare information relating to the following condition, treatment and dates:
All healthcare information:
Other:
Yes: _____ No: _____

I authorize the release of my STD/HIV/AIDS results whether negative or positive to the
Above named person. Yes: _____ No: _____

I authorize the release of any record regarding drug, alcohol or mental treatment to the
Above named person.

Patient Signature		Date Signed	

This authorization expires ninety days after it is issued.

Medical Release	
Patient's name	Date of Birth
Previous name	Social Security number

I request and authorize _____ to release healthcare information of The above named patient.		
Name		Address
City	State	Zip code
This request and authorization applies to _____		
Healthcare information relating to the following condition, treatment and dates: All healthcare information: Other: Yes: _____ No: _____		
I authorize the release of my STD/HIV/AIDS results whether negative or positive to the Above named person. Yes: _____ No: _____		
I authorize the release of any record regarding drug, alcohol or mental treatment to the Above named person.		
Patient Signature		Date Signed	
This authorization expires ninety days after it is issued.		

www.ingramcontent.com/pod-product-compliance
Lightning Source LLC
Chambersburg PA
CBHW081118180526
45170CB00008B/2903